Coconut Oil: Dispelling the Myths

The Numerous Uses of Coconut Oil

By: Raj Bennett

PUBLISHERS NOTES

Disclaimer

This publication is intended to provide helpful and informative material. It is not intended to diagnose, treat, cure, or prevent any health problem or condition, nor is it intended to replace the advice of a physician. No action should be taken solely on the contents of this book. Always consult your physician or qualified health-care professional on any matters regarding your health before adopting any suggestions in this book or drawing inferences from it.

The author and publisher specifically disclaim all responsibility for any liability, loss or risk, personal or otherwise, which is incurred as a consequence, directly or indirectly, from the use or application of any contents of this book.

Any and all product names referenced within this book are the trademarks of their respective owners. None of these owners have sponsored, authorized, endorsed, or approved this book.

Always read all information provided by the manufacturers' product labels before using their products. The author and publisher are not responsible for claims made by manufacturers.

Large Print Edition

Manufactured in the United States of America

DEDICATION

This book is dedicated to my parents and my loving wife Sandhya. Without their love and support and constant encouragement, I would not have been able to write, much less publish this book.

TABLE OF CONTENTS

PUBLISHERS NOTES 2
DEDICATION 3
TABLE OF CONTENTS 4
CHAPTER 1- WHAT IS COCONUT OIL AND HOW IS IT MADE? 5
CHAPTER 2- THE ADVANTAGES OF USING COCONUT OIL 13
CHAPTER 3- THE TYPES OF COCONUT OIL AND HOW THEY ARE PROCESSED 20
CHAPTER 4- HOW COCONUT OIL HELPS TO MAINTAIN THE SKIN 28
CHAPTER 5- HOW COCONUT OIL HELPS WITH HAIR CARE 35
CHAPTER 6- HOW COCONUT OIL HELPS TO HEAL THE BODY 42
CHAPTER 7- 10 COMMON MYTHS ABOUT COCONUT OIL 49
ABOUT THE AUTHOR 57

Raj Bennett

Chapter 1 - What Is Coconut Oil and How Is It Made?

The coconut is one of nature's powerhouse plants. It yields great benefits for health when its' oil and meat are used either internally or externally. The oil can be used as a lubricant in many ways and offers its own terrific benefits for the body.

Coconut Oil

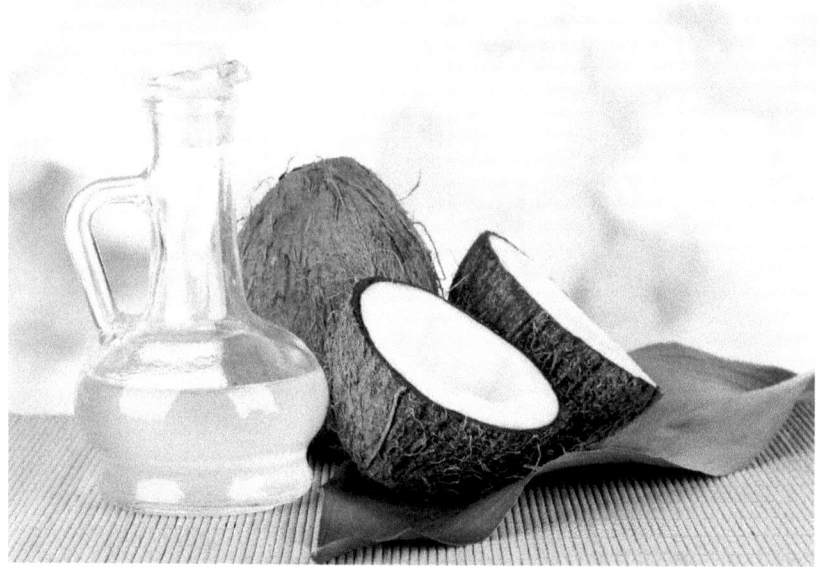

Most people are familiar with the coconut itself. A hard -shelled item that is not easily broken. Inside is the meat and milk. The coconut when split open yields the tasty treat from inside. The meat of the coconut can be eaten as it is, or dried before eating. It can be safely stored for later use. The dried meat is known as copra. The milk is good to drink and contains many vital nutrients. The real prize from the coconut is the oil it contains.

The meaty part of the coconut is dried and the oil extracted from the resulting copra. The drying process and extraction yields oil which is not yet food grade. In order to become food grade oil, a refining process takes place next. The refining of the oil removes some of the coconut flavor from it. This is a benefit for those who use it to cook.

Coconut milk yields the coconut oil and it must be separated in order to obtain the oil alone. This is easily done by pouring the milk into a container and covering it. It is then set aside where it will separate into a curd and a liquid. The liquid oil will remain in that state at temperatures over 76 degrees. Below that temperature, it will harden into a firm gel-like solid.

Once thought to be bad for the heart, coconut oil has since proven itself through nutritional research to be a superfood. Vegans have relied on this oil for years as a staple for cooking. It replaced butter and margarine in the vegan diet. Recent studies have shown that the saturated fats in coconut oil are beneficial to the cardio vascular system, dispelling the earlier negative opinions as myth.

Coconut oil contains Lauric acid which acts to raise the human blood levels of HDL or good cholesterol, an important substance for heart health. The coconut and its oil have been found to have many medicinal properties and as such have helped with:

- Controlling Viruses that cause flu and other diseases.
- Killing harmful bacteria that can cause many diseases including pneumonia.
- Driving out tapeworms and parasites from the body
- Repairing the skin when applied topically.
- Prevents aging of the body by strengthening the bones, supporting the heart and arterial system and works as

- an antioxidant. It has also been known to support brain health.
- When topically applied, it offers excellent benefits for the skin.

Coconut oil is simply different from other food-grade oils. The saturated fat in the oil has medium chain triglycerides which are highly beneficial to humans, unlike the longer chain fats found in almost all edible oils and plants.

Many users will take coconut oil directly by swallowing a tablespoon full at a time. Others will add the oil to their food when cooking or pour in coffee or other hot drinks. It can be used for frying at high temperatures and gives fried foods a unique taste.

The acceptance of coconut oil back into the dietary mainstream has been a long time coming. Due to pressure from large agricultural companies and major food processing companies, coconut oil was driven from the stores. The more profitable oils from corn and soy quickly grew in popularity. Their usage nationwide grew too as the public was misinformed about the benefits of these oils and the supposed harmful effects of coconut.

In recent years the turnabout has been tremendous and the many millions of coconut oil users have reported the many previously mentioned benefits and many more. The latest research shows that people with the highest rate of coconut oil use have obtained maximized health. The combination of coconut oil and a healthy diet do amazing things for the body and mind.

The methods of refining the coconut oil are varied. Chemical extraction is a common method of refinement. This method involves the use of solvents to extract the oil. This method also increases the shelf-life of the product but does not offer the highest quality oil. When fresh coconut meat is used for extraction, the oil it produces is known as virgin oil. Exposed to minimal refining with little heat and with no chemicals, the virgin coconut oil is of the highest quality and offers the consumer the most benefit. The coconut meat used in this process is dried quickly and then pressed to produce oil.

Though there are no true industry standards for the labeling virgin when it relates to coconut oil, the taste, odor and overall quality of this oil is obvious to the user.

Virgin coconut oil can be made at home, but in today's food markets it can be easily obtained. The cost of coconut oil is typically higher than the soy and corn oils it competes with. The benefits are so many that the cost to the consumer is a secondary consideration. Where once coconut oil was thought to be harmful to the body, the research today simply overflows with praise for this food. The many thousands of uses for coconut oil in cooking and diet as well as the practical uses make it almost incomparable among the multitude of food grade oils available in the world today. Coconut oil is truly a miracle of nature. Chapter 3 will discuss the different types of coconut oil in greater detail.

Chapter 2 - The Advantages Of Using Coconut Oil

One of the reasons that coconut oil is considered a superfood is because of the numerous health benefits that it provide. The oil contains a unique blend of fatty acids that can benefit the body in several ways. Here are the top 12 health benefits of using coconut oil.

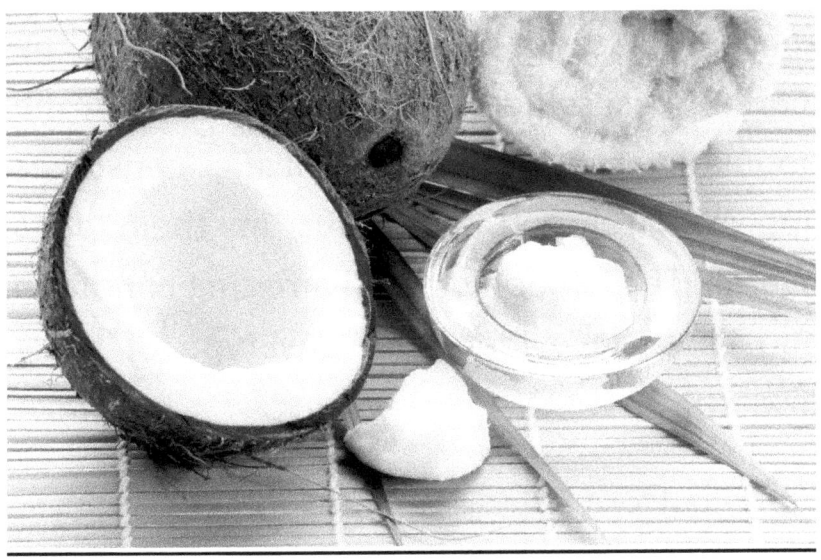

The Medicinal Properties Of Coconut Oil

The fatty acids in the coconut oil travel straight from the liver into the digestive tract.

Once the acids get into the digestive tract they are quickly turned into energy or into ketone bodies. The effects of the coconut oil can help with many disorders like Alzheimer's and brain disorders. The oil is metabolized differently helping to have a positive effect on different types of brain disorders.

Having A Healthier Body

Studies continue to show that people who consume coconut oil are the healthiest in the world. These studies go on to show how the population of the South Pacific consumes approximately 60% coconut in their diets overall. These people are in amazing condition and have no evidence of any type of heart disease.

Burning More Fat

The triglycerides in the coconut oil help to increase your energy levels. This in turn helps to burn fat at a faster rate. Consuming the coconut oil will give you a boost of approximately 5% compared to other foods, and will help you to lose significantly more weight in a shorter period of time.

Reduce Appearance Of Acne

The coconut oil can be applied topically to the skin to reduce the appearance of acne. The oils help to tighten and tone the outer layer of the skin, which can reduce the appearance of acne in a short time. The more tight and toned the skin's appearance, the more difficult it can be for acne to surface. In addition to a much clearer appearance, the skin will have a more supple and youthful glow.

Reduce Chapped Lips

The unique qualities of the coconut oil can protect the outer layer of skin on the lips. This coating can help to reduce chapped lips and protect the skin from the harmful rays of the sun. The coconut oil can be applied with a finger similar to applying a lip balm.

Fighting Off Bacteria

Coconut oil contains Lauric acid, which has a beneficial effect on killing bacteria, fungi, viruses, and infections. Over 50% of all the fatty acid in coconut oil is Lauric acid. When the coconut oil is digested, it can also form a Monolaurin. In combination with the Lauric acid, these two kill dangerous pathogens in the body that have an adverse effect on your body's health.

The Perfect Food Suppressant

One of the most difficult parts about losing weight is trying to curb your diet. The coconut oil helps to suppress your hunger and stop you from overeating without even trying. This is a huge benefit to people having difficulties staying on a diet. The long term effect of ingesting coconut oil is that you will eat less and be able to maintain your optimal body weight.

Reduce Seizures In The Body

Fatty acids from coconut oil can help to reduce seizures in the body. The coconut oil helps to increase ketone in the blood, which in turn has had significant positive effects on children suffering from epileptic seizures.

Improve Cholesterol Levels

Coconut contains an abundance of saturated fats which can help to lower your blood cholesterol levels. These saturated fats can help to lower the risk of heart disease as well. The coconut oil has been shown to also reduce triglycerides and improve the overall blood coagulation. These factors have been shown to reduce the risk of a potential heart attack or disease over the long term.

Coconut Oil
Protect And Moisturize The Skin

The unique qualities of coconut oil can help to moisturize the skin and help protect against sun damage. By increasing the lipid content in the skin, people who suffer from dry skin can benefit from a more supple and youthful appearance on the skin by applying the coconut oil directly to the body. The coconut oil has protective qualities that enable it to block 20% of the dangerous ultraviolet rays too. This makes it an effective sunscreen for the skin and the scalp. Using coconut oil topically is an effective way to fight off the aging properties of the sun, helping to protect the skin from sun spots and wrinkles.

Increase Brain Functions

The ketone produced by the coconut oil can help to provide the brain with alternative sources of energy. Studies have shown these ketone bodies have the ability to help lessen the symptoms associated with Alzheimer's.

Medium triglycerides have been shown in studies to give an immediate boost to the brain's functions in patients who were suffering with a mild form of the disease.

Reducing Dangerous Stomach Fat

The coconut oil has been shown in many studies to help reduce weight by increasing the ability to burn fat and to curb appetites. Another unique quality of coconut oil is it can also reduce the amount of abdominal fat in the body. The fat in the abdominal region is some of the most dangerous fats in the body. Coconut oil given to obese women was shown to reduce their BMI significantly in only 12 weeks. The same study showed even more significant results in men in much less time.

CHAPTER 3 - THE TYPES OF COCONUT OIL AND HOW THEY ARE PROCESSED

Coconuts thrive in areas where the sun is abundant, humidity is high and the rainfall is regular. Coconut trees are intolerant of cold weather and will thrive in tropical climates. In the United States, coconuts can be grown in Hawaii, southern Florida and the territories of American Samoa, Guam and Puerto Rico and the US Virgin Islands.

Coconut Oil

Coconut oil is extracted from the meat of a mature coconut harvested from a coconut palm tree. The oil has a high fat content, making it slow to oxidize and resistant to spoilage. Coconut oil can last as long as two years without becoming rancid. Health organizations advise against using too much coconut oil, no matter how it is processed, because of its high fat content.

Coconut oils have many uses and some types of oils have common uses, but the different coconut oils are not the same. Each of the different types of oils is better suited for different applications.

There are three basic types of coconut oil and include refined coconut oil, unrefined virgin coconut oil and hydrogenated coconut oil.

Refined Coconut Oil

As mentioned in Chapter 1, refined coconut oil is extracted from fresh coconut meat and with no chemical process involved, the oil is colorless, but has a mild and natural taste and odor. Refined coconut oil is made from dried coconut meat, called copra. The copra is placed in a hydraulic press and with the addition of heat the oil is extracted. The yield is about 60% of the dry weight of the coconut. Refined coconut oil is used in cooking and baking.

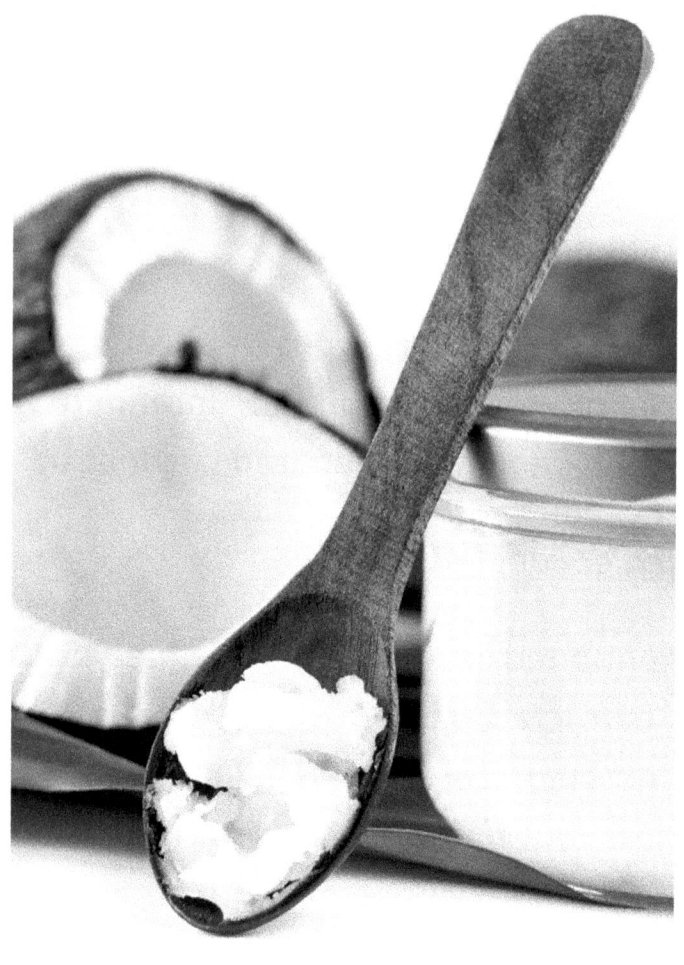

Unrefined Virgin Coconut Oil

Unrefined virgin coconut oil is the most natural and purest form of coconut oil and it looks almost as clear as water, as it is not changed with a heating process. This type of coconut oil is extracted from dried coconut meat or coconut milk and refined, bleached and deodorized to make it tasteless, odorless and colorless. The coconut oil is extracted using a screw press and grating it to a moisture content of 10 to 12 %. An additional press method is used to extract the oil. To produce oil from the coconut milk involves letting the milk ferment for 36 to 48 hours and separating the oil from the milk residue. The leftover cream can be heated and the milk will evaporate leaving any additional oil. Unrefined virgin coconut oil is used in lotions and soaps, massage oil, body and hair treatments, dietary supplement, syrups and smoothies.

Hydrogenated Coconut Oil

Hydrogenated coconut oil is injected with hydrogen gas at high pressure to up its melting point; this prolongs its shelf life. The oil converts good fatty acids to Tran's fatty acids that contribute to heart disease. This type of coconut oil is used widely as a food additive. Hydrogenated oil of any kind should be avoided.

The Oil Removal Process

There are two types of processes used to extract oil from coconut. The type of process used dictates the type of oil as a result. There are variations within each process to increase the yield of the oil in comparison to the volume of coconut meat. A rule of thumb for determining the amount of coconut oil is it takes approximately 1,000 mature coconuts that have a total weight of approximately 3,200 pounds will yield about 370 pounds of copra which yields about 18 US gallons of oil.

The Dry Process

The dry process requires the meat to be separated from the shell and then dried using kiln, sunlight or fire. The dried meat is called copra. The copra is then dissolved or pressed with solvents that produce coconut oil and a coconut mash that is high in fiber and protein. The mash is not of a quality for human consumption, but is used to feed to camels, giraffes, elk, deer, buffalo, bison, goats, sheep and cattle.

The Wet Process

The wet process uses fresh coconut meat rather than copra. The protein in the coconut creates an emulsion of water and oil and the difficult part is breaking up the emulsion to recover the oil. Modern wet process technologies include centrifugal force and a pretreatment system utilizing heat, cold, salts, acids, electrolysis, enzymes, shockwaves or some combination of them. However, the wet process delivers a 10 to 15% more yield than the dry process.

Coconut Oil
Home Made Coconut Oil

It is possible to make coconut oil at home by scraping the meat of the coconut and giving it a fine chop. Place the chopped coconut in a food processor and blend until the coconut is shredded using a medium speed. Place a small amount of shredded coconut in a piece of cheesecloth or coffee filter and squeeze the liquid into a jar. After all the coconut meat has been through the squeezing process, cover the jar and let it set for at least 24 hours. The coconut milk and oil will separate as the liquid sets and a layer of curd will appear at the top of the jar. The jar can be left in the refrigerator or a cool room. Remove the curd from the top of the jar and virgin coconut oil will remain in the jar.

Another method, using the wet process, is to heat 4 cups of water until it starts to steam. Grate the meat from two mature coconuts and place it into a blender along with the hot water. Puree the contents until the liquid becomes a smooth mixture. Place a piece of cheesecloth over a bowl and pour the blender contents over the cloth and let the mixture drip into the bowl. Using a spatula, squeeze the mixture through the cloth to get as much liquid as possible. Boil the liquid from the bowl until the water has evaporated and the cream has separated from the oil. Strain the oil from the liquid.

Chapter 4 - How Coconut Oil Helps To Maintain The Skin

In an effort to get beautiful skin; healthy and clear, many people not only try multiple products that don't really work for them, but can spend a fortune in their quest. But did you know that something as simple as coconut oil can be great for the skin, eliminating such things as acne while rejuvenating, nourishing, and replenishing moisture?

Coconut oil is also known for its healing and protecting properties that can have your skin looking more youthful, and more vibrant than you've seen it look in years. Maybe ever. Coconut oil helps to rectify dry and cracked areas. It will help to strengthen underlying, connective tissue, so that fine lines are no longer visible or noticeable. Instead, your skin will look fresh, and with little signs of aging.

Something many people want is to regain their youthful glow. Have you ever wished you could get back the youthful skin you once had, but over the years, it seems to have vanished? Maybe it was replaced by drier, more cracked and damaged skin.

Have you ever wished you could find a product that would help bring back all the positive attributes of your skin that it once had? Well, you can, and it's as easy as using a simple product - coconut oil. Coconut oil is an all-natural product that has multiple benefits for the skin. It's great for all of your skin, but for your facial skin, it can bring back its younger, more vibrant appearance.

Some of the most beneficial properties of coconut oil that help to achieve younger, fresher skin are:

- It is a facial skin highlighter - Did you know that if you brush on a small amount of coconut oil on top of your make-up, then let it dry, your skin will glow and instantly look more vibrant and alive? Coconut oil is a natural

luminizer; highlighting your natural pigment tones.
- It is packed with anti-microbial properties – As you saw in chapter one, one of the most effective properties of coconut oil is the fact that it contains medium-chain fatty acids. These fatty acids are known for their anti-microbial properties. These anti-microbial properties help to alleviate viruses, fungi and bacteria, to give you clean, fresh, and healthy skin.
- It is a deep, skin conditioner - Coconut oil is one of the best conditioners there is for skin. It helps to not only cleanse, but also soothe many conditions of the skin. Some of the most common skin conditions that coconut oil can help relieve and alleviate are:
    - Acne
    - Athlete's foot
    - Ringworm

- Thrush
- Skin rashes; such as, diaper rash
- Jock itch

If you could find a skin product that not only helps relieve certain skin conditions, but makes your skin glow, was all-natural with no harsh chemicals, and didn't leave a residue or feel greasy, wouldn't you want to use it? Well, that is exactly what coconut oil is. Being that it is all-natural, you won't have any of the side-effects you get with a lot of products. Some products may help with one issue, but cause others; such as skin redness and irritation. They may clog pores and cause skin breakouts, with blackheads and blemishes. Some products can even burn the skin, leaving it red, irritated and sensitive. With coconut oil, you don't have to worry about any of that. Coconut oil is pure, and gentle to even the most sensitive skin.

Coconut Oil

Coconut oil is mostly fats, which means it is full of emollients. Emollients are soothing to the skin and can bring a lot of relief to many skin issues. Emollients also create softer skin, which is just one way it helps blemishes to heal quickly, and thoroughly. And because coconut, like other skin creams and treatments, is absorbed into the lymphatic system, it works from the inside out, but it is safe and natural. Knowing it is so pure, should make you feel good about using such a safe product on your skin.

Do you have fine lines? Most people get them around their eyes, their mouth, even on the forehead and cheeks. Coconut oil strengthens the connective tissue that gives skin its suppleness, elasticity and flexibility. Giving your skin its strength back will help to reduce the appearance of fine lines. It will help to eliminate dead skin cells, which means a reduction in skin flaking. Your skin will look and feel smooth. It will glow.

When it comes to treating acne, what is the best way to use it to get the most benefits? The best way is to first, steam your face. This helps to open the pores so the coconut oil gets deep into each pore. Once you've steamed and opened your pores, apply a thin layer of the oil on your skin and allow it to stay on for 2 minutes; then gently wipe it off. You don't want it to sit on the skin too long, or it also can clog the pores and cause your acne problem to worsen, like any other product.

Although coconut oil is pure, you should always give it a test run on your skin, just in case. Make sure you don't have any sensitivities or reactions. To do a trial run, first, apply a small amount on the area you want to treat. Allow it to sit there a couple of minutes, and then wipe it off. If you do not notice any type of redness, or burning effect, then you can apply the full amount all over the area you want to treat.

Coconut Oil

Coconut oil is also inexpensive. A whole bottle will last months and months. How many products can you say that about?

Chapter 5 - How Coconut Oil Helps With Hair Care

If you find that you have damaged or brittle hair you will likely want to try to find something that will address this. There are a full range of coconut oil treatments that people can use to repair the damage that they have sustained. But it will be important for people to think about some of the different treatments that they can use. Combining different products can be an excellent method of getting the perfect look for hair in just a short amount of time. you will likely appreciate a rundown of the different products containing coconut oil out on the market. They can often be used in conjunction with other treatments, improving the results that you may see for yourself.

Coconut Oil

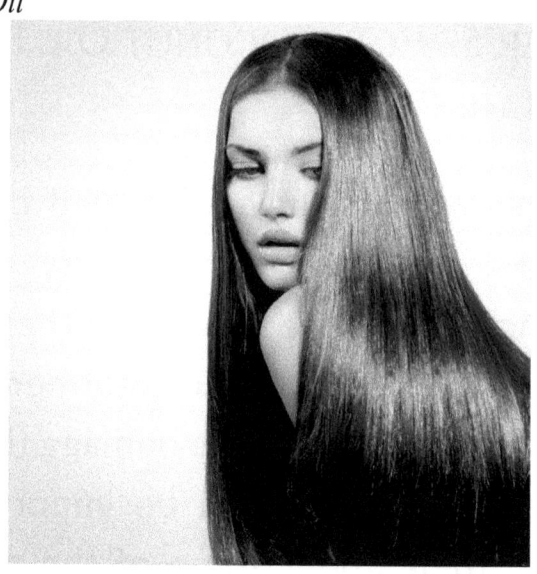

You may be interested in learning how you can actually apply pure coconut oil to your hair. This is becoming increasingly popular, thanks to the fact that coconut oil is becoming more readily available. Coconut oil can be bought from a supplier who will be able to help people improve the look to their hair. This oil can be difficult to use and it may be messy when applying it to hair. This is part of the reason why you will want to think about boosting the quality of your hair over time. Consumers should think about applying the coconut oil in the shower, which will help them contain the way that it is applied. They can even set down newspaper to help protect appliances and fixtures during this process.

Though you won't have to do it every day, you should think about applying coconut oil fairly regularly. This could be an invaluable asset for you if you want to improve your look in just a short amount of time. The more frequently it is applied, the more easily it can be used to enhance the overall quality of hair. You will appreciate that your hair will just be more durable after this kind of treatment. This will help you get the look that you want to see and even helps you style you're hair however you may want. Hair treated with coconut oil will tend to be more durable and will stand up to different types of chemical applications.

There are actually quite a few different types of specialty treatments that will utilize coconut oil. This product can be used to help people specialize the deep conditioning treatment that they want to get. Deep conditioning treatment can be used to apply coconut oil directly to the scalp as well. People can then massage it in and get even better results for themselves. This could be the perfect solution for the quality of their hair over time. The oil itself can blend down in to the roots of hair follicles that they want to improve. This could be an invaluable asset for people who just want longer and more luxurious hair. Many hair stylists are looking for ways that they can integrate this treatment in to their services, since it does provide some impressive results.

People with specific hair problems may actually be able to get some support from the treatments that they decide to use. There are many different types of detanglers that can be used to improve the overall texture of hair. But consumers are starting to wonder how they can improve on the basic results of the treatment that they want to see. If you are searching for a sleeker texture for their hair, you will likely want to think about how this oil may work. There are actually shampoos that are being specifically designed to feature this oil, which will be an invaluable consideration for you to remember.

Dandruff treatment is often an invaluable asset for most people to consider, since it will improve the look of their hair. Coconut oil is a great resource for people who want to cut down on the flakes that they see. The oil should be applied on a fairly regular basis, since it will be helping to moisturize the scalp. Many people suffer from dandruff when their skin tends to dry out excessively. It will be important for people to consider how dry skin can be impacted by some of these different types of products over time as well.

If consumers don't want the hassle of pure coconut oil, they do have other options. Many different hair care treatment products are starting to offer people the opportunity to buy it at the market. There are many new conditioners and shampoos that incorporate coconut oil into their formulas. Think about how you can review the listing of the ingredients that the companies tend to use over time. This could be an important consideration if you need to improve on the basic results that you want to see as well. You should try making sure that you are buying products that will contain authentic coconut oil.

Reading through consumer reviews can actually be an indispensable resource for many out on the market. This can help you adjust to the basic techniques that you may use throughout the day as well. There are actually several packages that will put together everything that you need to get the perfect look for yourself. Some customers may want to check reviews to make sure all the ingredients are safe. This is particularly important for people who want to avoid having any kind of allergic reaction. In the next chapter you will see how coconut oil can help other areas of the body.

Chapter 6- How Coconut Oil Helps To Heal The Body

Usually when we think about products with fats such as coconut oil, we consider them to be unhealthy and to be bad for our hearts. Through studies we have come to learn that coconut oil does not fit that way of conventional thinking. In fact, coconut oil is actually considered a heart-healthy supplement that aids your body in several ways.

Coconut Oil in a "Nutshell"

Coconut oil in its purest form can be found bearing a label that shows it is virgin and organic, this is when it contains no hydrogenation and has 92% saturated fat. This is the highest amount found in any fat. When held at room temperature, a saturated fat will become solid. These are usually found in animal products such as meat or dairy products and have high cholesterol in them.

When tropical oil is held at room temperatures, instead of just becoming solid, its form can vary anywhere from a solid to a liquid state. Also unlike animal fats, tropical oil fats do not contain cholesterol. Several researchers also suggest that using coconut oil in moderation can give your body added benefits from the possible plant chemicals that are absorbed.

Similar to fats, coconut oils contain a combination of different fatty acids. The unusual blend found specifically in coconut oil is thought to be the source of these benefits. Coconut oil contains four primary medium to short chain fatty acids: lauric, caprylic, myristic, and capric. These particular fatty acids are metabolized rapidly and will give you a great natural boost of energy instead of being held in your body as fat.

Calorically, coconut oil still has the same amount of calories per gram as other fats do. A single tablespoon bears 117 calories and will contribute 14 grams of fat with 12 grams saturated fat. It also will not provide any vitamins or minerals. However, its high smoke point gives foods a wonderful tropical flavor, makes it resistant to burning, and since it has no carbs, it is also terrific as cooking oil.

Immunity Benefits

Recent studies have been done to help support the benefits of taking coconut oil daily as a health supplement. These studies show that ingesting it can help the body's resistance to many viruses and bacteria. It has been effective in fighting yeast and fungal infections.

Coconut oil also benefits the control of blood sugar through its ability to help improve insulin levels. It also allows your thyroid to increase in function giving your metabolism, endurance, and strength a boost. Coconut also has the ability to help you absorb fat soluble vitamins, rapidly aiding your digestion.

Coconut Oil And Cholesterol

Specifically, lauric acid found in coconut oil holds benefits to helping cholesterol levels. Lauric acid is a type of medium-chain triglyceride (MCT). MCT's are easily metabolized and absorbed by your body. It can increase your energy. Lauric acid also helps increase your HCL or "good" cholesterol to improve healthy cholesterol ratios. An improperly functioning thyroid can lead to imbalanced hormones and high cholesterol levels. Since coconut oil also has the ability to help balance these hormones, it in turn lowers bad cholesterol levels.

Weight Management

As stated in chapter 2, medium chain triglycerides are found in coconut fat. These MCT's are considered healthy fats because of their ability to be easily broken down by your body. When these fats are proficiently broken down by your liver you will also burn energy more efficiently. This ability to burn energy effectively will then alleviate the stress put on your pancreas in turn increasing your metabolic rate and reducing fat accumulation.

Anti-Aging Properties

Oxidation is thought to be the primary culprit in the breakdown of healthy tissue which contributes to aging seen overtime in your skin as well as cardiovascular deterioration. In order to counteract this process, our bodies need to take in more antioxidants. Coconut oil has good anti-oxidant levels that can help prevent oxidation to the healthy fat and tissue in our bodies.

Benefits To Skin And Hair

Similar to mineral oil, coconut oil is an effective moisturizer when massaged into the skin. However, unlike mineral oils, coconut oil does not have unfavorable side effects, making it much safer for treating dry and flaking skin. You can find coconut oil in many skin care products that are used to treat skin conditions such as psoriasis, dermatitis, and eczema since it also has a high amount of vitamin E which defends the skin. Coconut oil is even safe and gentle enough for protecting infant skin and can be massaged into your baby's skin after a warm bath without any adverse side effects.

Other Health Benefits

Coconut oil has been suggested as a benefit for many other ailments. Though it will not cure the following issues, it has been found that coconut oil has a proven mild benefit in their treatment.

Kidney Function: Aids in dissolving kidney stones and prevention of kidney and gall bladder issues.

Stress Relief: Aromatherapy shows coconut oil to be helpful in alleviating stress through the application of the oil to your temples.

Bone Benefits: Coconut oils allow bones to absorb needed minerals including calcium and magnesium which are imperative for bone health including teeth.

Side Effects

When taken in moderate amounts, coconut oils are thought to be very safe with no side effects. The suggested daily dose for maximum benefits is two tablespoons. Studies are still being conducted to legitimize claims but the potential benefits of coconut oil seems to abound showing positive effects on many body systems, thyroid issues, weight management, and heart disease.

CHAPTER 7- 10 COMMON MYTHS ABOUT COCONUT OIL

It's easy enough to follow the hype on all these diet fads obediently without giving any of them so much as a quick read up on all that they're about, but now it's time to get educated about the things you're putting into your body or plan to consume. With every fad there are myths and there are truths. And though it's not the latest fad, coconut oil is still getting a lot of attention by health nuts, medical professionals, and the average Joe. So, in honor of this natural oil that so many people call the best alternative to greasy butters and fattening oils, I've put together the top ten myths to help entertain your mind about your body. There are two different kinds of myths. There are myths that present the topic at hand as being good and positive and miraculous, and a perfect investment. And then then there are myths that present the topic at hand as being dumb and bad and a waste of time and money. As this book is meant to be unbiased, I will be presenting you with both types so you can get all the facts and make up your mind about it for yourself.

Myth Number One: "Coconut oil is the healthiest oil I can have."

Fact: Even though it is cholesterol-free, coconut oil is still a saturated fat which means that it must be limited in one's diet. The best alternative is to use vegetable oils. Extra virgin olive oil is said by medical professionals to be the healthiest type of oil.

Myth Number Two: "Being allergic to coconuts means that I can't use coconut oil."

Fact: The allergy to coconuts is based on the incapability to digest its proteins. The coconut's proteins are located in the meat of the tropical nut and not the oil. Because of this, one can use coconut oil even if they are allergic to the nut.

Myth Number Three: "Because coconut oil is a saturated fat, prolonged use means I'm risking heart disease and heart failure."

Fact: Heart disease and heart failure have never been provably connected to the use of coconut oil. The base for this myth is 100% presumptuous and has no strong data to back up such hazardous claims.

Myth Number Four: "Only virgin coconut oil is healthy for me; refined coconut oil is horrible."

Fact: Though no form of coconut oil is the healthiest choice, all types of coconut oil are considered "healthy" options. Virgin coconut oil is better for you than refined coconut oil, but neither is particularly unhealthy.

Myth Number Five: "Coconut oil prevents Alzheimer's disease."

Fact: The theory about coconut oil helping Alzheimer's is based on the concept that the ketone bodies inside of the coconut oil can present different energy sources to brain cells that have grown incapable of utilizing glucose because of the Alzheimer's disease. However, though there have been studies that give the allure of that possibility, there's absolutely no conclusive proof that coconut oil can or cannot help people suffering from Alzheimer's disease.

Myth Number Six: "Because coconut oil is composed of saturated fats, consuming it will make me gain weight and lead to obesity."

Fact: Coconut oil has medium fatty acids which actually aid in speeding up the metabolism. Believe it or not, coconut oil is even prescribed by some physicians as a potential way to lose weight.

Myth Number Seven: "Coconut oil is going to make my skin irritated."

Fact: Not only is this myth incorrect, but like many others, the truth is the exact opposite. Coconut oil is actually commonly prescribed as a skin soother. It can also make a great exfoliant when mixed with certain other natural fruits and herbs. Coconut oil is also said to help plaque psoriasis, and eczema and can keep it under control and prevent further breakouts.

Myth Number Eight: "It's not easily absorbed into the skin."

Fact: Though most pictures of coconut oil make it seem incredibly thick, it is actually a very thin oil and absorbs quickly into the skin, in fact, it is often preferred to most massage and tanning oils.

Myth Number Nine: "Coconut oil is sweet and bad for diabetics."

Fact: Just because coconuts are sweet, everyone assumes that coconut oil is sweet as well: but it actually has little to no flavor whatsoever. Also, coconut oil helps the body secrete insulin from the pancreas, so it's not only a completely false myth, but it actually winds up helping diabetics.

Myth Number Ten: "Coconut oil goes rancid way too easily."

Fact: To the contrary, coconut oil is one of the longest lasting oils due to it containing more moisture than admissible. In fact, as mentioned in chapter 4, it has one of the longest shelf lives of all oils.

Raj Bennett

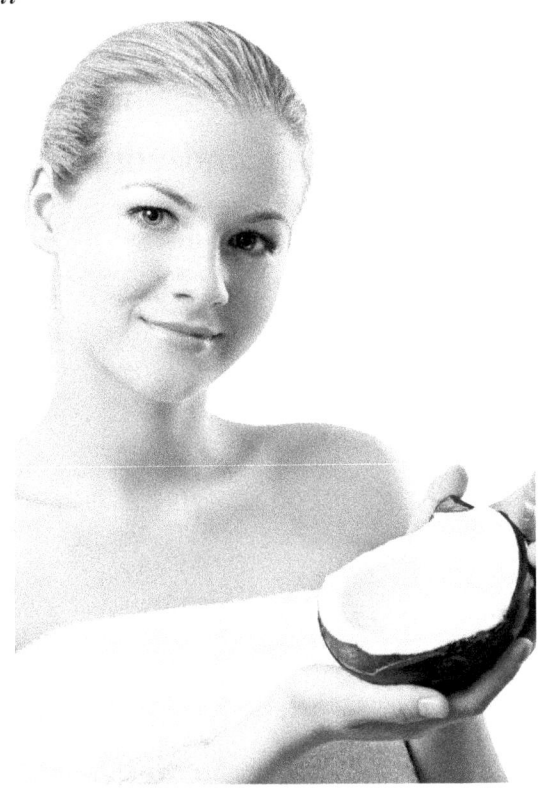

Not everyone wants to do the research to expose the lies and distinguish the myths from the facts. That's where I come in. So there you have it, now that you have a clear list of the ten most common myths about coconut oil and the facts that debunk them all, hopefully, you've learned something about this tropical nut's natural oils and about not believing everything you hear. I'm sure it will be easier for you to decide whether or not you want to get into the habit of using coconut oil for yourself and your family now that you've heard the truth.

About The Author

Raj Bennett grew up in a household where he was encouraged to research and find out more information about anything that he was interested in (within reason of course). As a result of this he spent quite a lot of time doing research on things he had questions about and finding out if the information that he had received prior to about a particular topic, like coconut oil, was really valid.

He carried this zeal for research into his adult life and even when he got married; his wife did not discourage him from doing his research. In fact, she was happy to support him as he would never fail to support her when necessary.

Raj's family all uses coconut oil daily and enjoy the many benefits that could be gained from its daily use.

www.ingramcontent.com/pod-product-compliance
Ingram Content Group UK Ltd.
Pitfield, Milton Keynes, MK11 3LW, UK
UKHW022219230426
12048UKWH00016BA/934